Joe Collins

FROM
DARK NIGHTS
TO
BRIGHTER DAYS

This book is published by LMD Publications.
Book ISBN: 978-1-9162296-3-1

LMD Publications

Contents

I dedicate this book to all of the people out there that
are suffering from mental health issues.
I know first-hand, how dark life can get.
There is hope and there is light at the end of the tunnel.
Stay positive, stay strong.

Chapter 1
My Story

The main challenge I have had to face within my life started one Saturday night in May 2012. It would, being honest with myself, take until the beginning of 2020 to get me out of the mess I let myself get into just from this one incident.

Up until this point, I had the world at my feet, with a signed professional contract with Warrington Wolves. This was the year after having amazing success going undefeated through my last year of school and amateur rugby at under 16's.

The Ince Rose Bridge team I played for was littered with up-and-coming stars, with seven of us signing professional contracts. I personally had only started playing rugby two years before this and got picked up by Warrington Wolves to join their scholarship system. I wasn't a very gifted rugby player, but I had some strengths that worked in my favour. I was very lucky to have a dad who pushed to me to play all kinds of sports and would drive me around everywhere. He also raised me to be very disciplined, taking me to the gym to go on the punch bags and lift weights, because at the time - he felt I was a bit soft and he was probably right.

Dad brought me up to take on the world, never take a backward step and never be scared of anything. The one thing I feared however was letting him down, because if I didn't give 100% at something, he would come down on me like a tonne of bricks. By the time I left school, my fitness, physical toughness and aggression had led to me gaining a lot of success. Especially in the sporting world winning the league, National Cup and County Cup with Rose Bridge and the North West Counties Cup with school and just missing out in the National Schools final, where I was captain.

 My dad had brought me up to play on the edge and not back down from anyone. If somebody gave me any grief, I had to run straight at them with the ball with all my aggression. There was no side stepping or passing, even though I was 3-4 stone lighter than most prop forwards. It was about being fearless because that's who I was brought up to be.

It was great at the time. Everyone loved playing and training with me because of the high standards and work ethic I'd been brought up with, but one incident one night changed all of that. When we reached 16 years of age, the Rose Bridge team that hadn't lost all season, went its separate ways to professional clubs. Like I said before, I had come into the game and got asked to go to Warrington which I was really pleased with. As a 16-year-old, after leaving school, I started getting paid to play and train for Warrington Wolves. The first pre-season and first month of the season couldn't have gone better. I was awarded the *"Player of the Month"* and consolidated my place in the starting team after starting the first game on the bench. The future looked ridiculously bright and I loved it there.

Over my time at Rose Bridge, the lads there were my best friends, my brothers. I would have run through a brick wall for them and I hoped that despite us coming to play against each other, that things would stay the same.

Unexpectedly, things changed almost instantly. The atmosphere amongst us had grown sour. I was going to Warrington training and rumours about me were flying about from the lads at Wigan. Silly little rumours, but the atmosphere had changed, and I gathered that they simply didn't want to associate with me anymore. I could not understand why this had happened and what the need for it was. I decided to confront one of them about the situation which got slightly heated, but the moment had passed by and I thought nothing of it. That was until one summer night in Wigan town centre when the full Wigan team was out. I was also out with some friends who were just quiet lads. They weren't into rugby, just normal lads who enjoyed a bit of sport and a drink at the weekend.

The next thing I know, the Wigan lads were up in my face giving me all sorts of abuse in numbers - I found this hard. I was brought up never to take a backwards step from anyone. I knew going head-to-head over a drunken argument and some petty things wasn't a good idea. Not only that, but I was also only 17, so I shouldn't have been out drinking really. A few of my mates ushered me away. We said we would go to a club at the other side of Wigan, which we thought was a sensible idea. When walking to this nightclub, suddenly, I felt a whack to the back of my head. Then they raised my t-shirt over my head locking my arms up so I couldn't use them, and I couldn't see. I was getting laid into big time from a few of them. I couldn't shake them off me with my shirt over my head, so I took to trying to morally bring them down shouting, *"is this all you've got?"* It carried on for no more than a couple of minutes. I fell and it came to the lowest point of a friend, who I played rugby for years, hitting me whilst I was on the floor and jumping up cheering like he had won the World Cup. I was down but luckily not too injured - just a bit of a bruise on one of my eyes. A few of my friends from the night helped to break it up and bring the fight to an end. Physically, it had not done much damage. All the years of weights and rugby had worked to my advantage. I was lucky really, one wrong landing for me and it could have been potentially very dangerous. Physically, I was fine, but emotionally I was hurt big time.

This story isn't to blame anyone or get my revenge. Everyone makes mistakes in this life; everyone does stupid things sometimes and hurts people. No matter how nice you are, it's just part of the growing process. Life is one big lesson and we are constantly learning and making mistakes and it seems in life we only learn the hard way, never the easy way, no matter how hard we try. This story is about me and how poorly I dealt with it. How I let my anger from this situation lead to me self-sabotaging my rugby career and my life to the point where I self- destructed. I am lucky by the grace of God to still be here to tell this story.

So, the question now was how did I handle what had happened to me? Did I do what my nature had been to do for all of my rugby days and go and face them head on? This would mean risking my rugby career that I had worked so hard for. After much consideration, I decided that one day I would get my shot at redemption on the pitch - so I would wait until then.

Looking back, neither of the solutions were a good idea. It let the anger fester in me. Every day, I thought about getting my payback. Each time I lifted a weight – I pictured them. The anger made me super strong, but that kind of motivation isn't healthy, you can't just get rid of it after training. I also, after that night, should never have had a drink or entered Wigan town centre on a night out again. It wasn't good for me.

Alcohol is a depressant and when you're angry inside, it's

toxic for you. I used to go out most Saturday nights and stay out until 6am, trying to make myself feel better. Drinking too much to keep myself calm because in my head, there was always a chance it could happen again. I was starting to feel depressed. I was still training and playing rugby, but my standards had started to slip. I wasn't focused enough on each game. All I focused on was playing against Wigan and getting my revenge. Throughout that time, all that was going through my head was, *"Who do they think they are? How could they do that to me? I'm going to destroy them! They won't stand a chance!"*

I wasn't training for the next game, I just trained for the day I got to face them. Maybe my dreams of playing for the first team had gone. Now I was just focussed on paying them back, feeding my own ego and making them regret their actions from that awful night.

In the meantime, I was telling my parents how low I was feeling, but then going out until 6am every Saturday drinking. I thought it was okay because it was the only time that I felt happy, because the alcohol numbed my pain. My dad always said to me, I wasn't any good when I was tired, and he was right. The nights out and my attitude were the problem. If I would have stopped drinking then and got some counselling, I know the problems would have ended -

but I didn't. I was 17 and what 17-year- old is going to stop drinking and hanging around with their mates on a Saturday night? Not many would have the strength to and neither did I.

We didn't play Wigan that season, but the following season the fixtures were announced, and we would play them on the second game. My chance had come, I had spent all of pre-season thinking about this. My friends at the time had even nicknamed it *"Judgement Day"*, like *The Terminator.*

My focus wasn't where it should have been in the pre-season either. I was still 3 stone lighter than most people in my position. I spent the pre-season angry and lifting too many weights, instead of focussing on my strength of being fitter than everyone else.

We played the first game of the season and I was shocking. I wasn't as fit as I used to be and we got beaten.
The following week, I got put on the bench for the Wigan game, which I deserved. This further fuelled my insecurities; I was so embarrassed which was making me even more psyched up. I had to win that game at all costs. Only one of the four lads involved in the incident that night was playing, but a lot of the other lads had since jumped on the bandwagon. I'd lost further friends, who had stopped talking

to me as soon as they'd signed their professional contract, which just fuelled my anger even more. I came off the bench and we were losing, but it was a close game. I was doing okay, making some decent runs but time was running out and we were still behind. I couldn't lose to Wigan after what had gone on. I took a carry on as hard as I could, the ball came out in contact and I knocked on. This grew my frustration. A few moments later, I aggressively shot out the defensive line to make a big hit on one of the opposition players. He decided to step to the side at the last minute, causing me to reach out with my arm, catch him on his chin and knock him flat out.

I got a straight red card and it got me in a lot of bother at Warrington. There was a picture taken of the tackle with my feet in the air whilst catching him on his chin. The caption of the picture that was going round on social media was, *"is this the worst high tackle you've ever seen?"* I got banned for a game or two for this. I felt so low, there was only me getting all this grief. There were other big lads in my team - they weren't getting the abuse off first teamers who were 10 years older than me. Why me? This also occurred in the gym whilst I was trying to train on a Saturday morning. It was also hard to escape these people, Wigan is a rugby town and the names of these people would be mentioned to me or I would hear their names every day.

Especially as their careers flourished, so I couldn't escape what had happened. What had I done to deserve this? It was challenging to say the least. For someone who had been taught to get fired up and just run over his problems and go head-to-head with anyone who had a problem with me. In hindsight, I should have handled it better, a lot better.

During the same time, I had opened up to my coaches about struggling mentally. My main coach was an old school, no nonsense type of guy and liked the way I played. He was always there for me, but the big wigs at the club didn't quite understand my strengths the same. After I had been sent off in the Wigan game and opened up about my struggles, one of them told me I wouldn't be able to go any further at the club with what I was going through. I couldn't believe what I was hearing. I believed and was told that you could now open up in sport after what happened to Terry Newton. Terry was a former Great Britain rugby league player who very sadly committed suicide. I was shocked to get this reaction and it added to my dismay and anger. After all, I had gone through all of this because I was a Wigan lad who had dared to sign for the arch enemy. Surely, I should have been understood more.

I'm telling this story, but I know now that it was all my fault. We make our own decisions; we choose our own habits.

That said, I do also believe that everything happens for a reason and everything is fated out. Nevertheless, I could have made my own life easier and at least made the most out of my rugby career by enjoying it, not feeling sorry for myself and making better, positive decisions. I don't blame anyone for the breakdown of my rugby career, it was all my own fault. I'm airing these things, so it doesn't happen again - to make life easier for people within the sport who are struggling and so that people think about taking the sport too far again. I hope people will think twice in future, because there's a lot more to life than sport even though we love it so much.

After my short ban, I came back and started playing a bit better. We had a good win against St Helens and I remember the coach, who I loved, saying to me that he had seen the old Joe Collins back on Saturday.
When I thought that things might be looking up, life decided to throw another challenge at me. The head coach who I loved was leaving and his assistant was taking over, who I'd never really bonded with. It became apparent that the big wigs at the top would now be having more control over the decisions and in his first game, I wasn't in the 18-man squad for the first time in my career. Even after playing well in a win against St Helens the week before. I was shocked at this and then again, I wasn't picked the following week or the

week after. In the space of 12 months, I'd gone from captaining the side for a game and being in the starting team every week, to not being able to get in the squad. What had happened to me?

A few weeks later, I finally got a chance to play again from the substitutes bench. I came on the pitch and played 10 minutes, made a few decent carries and got dragged off again. It was a bad day, nobody was playing well, but there were certainly a lot worse performances than me on that day. Yes, hand on heart I wasn't the fittest forward in the league, which I was the year before, but something just wasn't right, I was raging. I then got thrown on with 2 minutes to go in a match. I was defending when the opposing full back, one of the smaller faster players on the team broke through. I sprinted across and dived to tackle to avoid any further embarrassment. Unfortunately, I caught his chin and knocked him out cold. Another sending off, this time I got an 8-game ban. My Warrington career was basically done for. I never gained my spot back and spent the remaining part of the season playing water boy. As much as I didn't think so at the time, this was my fault. I'd let my anger from that night destroy my Warrington career. It was my fault, nobody else's. Even though I think the people at the club maybe could have helped me deal with my struggles better instead of telling me I couldn't go any further because I was depressed.

During this time, I started going to see the doctors to help me with how I was feeling. Unfortunately, this made me feel worse. All they did was push tablets down my throat which I didn't want to take because of the rugby, and they tried to diagnose me with different mental illnesses. This just made me feel alien and like there was no hope, when I know now, all I needed was counselling to help me work on getting rid of my anger and clear my head out to focus on doing what I loved. That wasn't an option though. I was told counselling didn't work very well with what I was going through. I didn't help myself again because I always felt sorry for myself and I wasn't very positive in trying to find a solution.

In the next season, I luckily got picked up by my old Rose Bridge coach to spend a year playing at Widnes Vikings. I knew he would get me back to my best and he did. There was no carrying too much weight around playing for him. I could tell he knew my strengths and would never be dishonest with me. He loved the way I played, and I would do anything for him as I owed my success so far in rugby to his coaching. The season was up and down throughout. I got back to my best and got my big win against Wigan, at Wigan, which was a great day and we beat most of the big teams like St Helens and Leeds.

I had a good season and played well in most games, but we could have done better overall, especially after beating the big teams. I thought I had done enough to earn a first team contract, but deep down I had a feeling it wasn't meant to be, and I was right. I was too old for the under-19s team and was released, but I had no regrets. This time I'd tried my best and could leave with my head held high.

At the time, I had just qualified as a personal trainer and was doing pretty well at it. I was looking forward to focussing solely on that. I'd spent most of my life in a gym and loved helping people, so it was perfect for me. I spent the next two years after playing rugby as a bit of a recluse, not really socialising or going out. Working 7 days a week. I was happy at work, but my emotions were still all over the place and in the summer of 2014, when I was at Widnes, I had encountered some family difficulties which led to me not speaking to my dad. He was doing his best, but it just wasn't what I needed at the time. I was constantly thinking about the old-school, no-nonsense upbringing he'd given me, and whether it had a link to why the Wigan lads did what they did because they didn't want to face me. I had started to wish I had chosen a different life rather than trying to be a physically tough, professional sportsman. This caused a lot of arguments between me and my dad. He was doing his best to help, by using his own strengths. My dad's strength isn't really his communication skills and he didn't really know how to sit down with me and talk about how I was feeling. He was understandably very worried about me, but at this time, I needed mellowing to calm me down as I was already angry enough. My work life was decent, I was earning good money, but my emotional problems were still unresolved. I hid away from them for a few years just working and avoided nights out mainly. This was until 2016. I had worked really hard in the gym and was in a bodybuilder shape. However, I was still training using anger as my motivation. Deep down I needed healing, but I thought I was okay at the time. Looking back, I realise now that all I wanted was to be loved, even though people did love me. I wanted to love myself, but I didn't. I hated myself for messing my rugby career up and for the stuff that had gone on with my dad. Dad and I never got the chance to sit down and talk to each other, leaving unresolved emotions to fester allowing my anger to flourish even more.

Since I had become so angry and been using the anger to lift really heavy weights, (being angry when lifting weights has been proven to increase the weights you can lift but running on that anger isn't good for you emotionally), my size had increased dramatically. This made me feel untouchable. I was filling my mind with stupid stuff, watching too much Danny Dyer's *Deadliest Men* and being obsessed with being hard like it was good thing. It was like my shield to protect myself from ever getting hurt again, without needing anyone to look up to.

I was about to learn the hard way. This behaviour was not a good way to live - I was in a trance of anger. I was back to drinking at the weekends. When I was on a night out, everyone wanted to be my friend because I was so big and they felt safe around me. I was hanging around with people who were in a real negative place and they were bigging up my confidence by wanting to hang around with me.

I felt unstoppable. I began to lose my morals, hanging round with these people who were in a negative head space. I started to follow their ways on nights out by taking drugs and thinking it was okay, thinking I was invincible. This carried on for a few months and it was fuelled by the fact that I never had to pay for any of it because I was big and people wanted me to hang round with them, so they felt safe. In this time, I also got jumped again because I wasn't acting like myself, being an idiot after a drink brought it on. Luckily, I had no real injuries, but this should have been the recurrence of an old wake-up call, but it wasn't. I was on the path to self- destruction.

One night, I got the biggest wake-up call to date. I was having a bad night. Somehow, I managed to lose all of my money during the night. This made me feel like shit and I already felt like I didn't have the confidence to go and enjoy my night. I hit rock bottom and took two pills to make myself feel better. After an hour or two, I felt really bad. I couldn't breathe, my heart was racing, and my chest was really tight - I thought I was dying. I even walked into Wigan hospital to get help. I luckily got told it was really busy and I decided to go for a walk instead. I thought my life was over, I couldn't get rid of this feeling, it was horrible. I thought I was going to die, luckily the fresh air pulled me around a bit and sobered me up.

It was the biggest wake-up call of my life. God had chosen to save me. Those two pills could have sent me to a very early grave. I was fuming with myself; I had woken up and thought, *"what the fuck am I doing? You could have had everything in your life, but you fucked it up."* I'd felt sorry for myself for too long, blaming it on the Wigan lads, blaming it on my dad. All of this anger had just nearly cost me my life and what was it all for? Idiot. I was thinking what a waste of life that would have been if I'd died. I've always been a big believer in God and believe to this day he decided to save me from that darkness because I still had work to do. So, I could tell this story, save as many people as possible and make the world a better place.

Thankfully on that night, I had just had a panic attack. I was fine, it was horrible though for the next 6 months. I struggled to comprehend what I had done. It was against everything that I believed in. How did I slip into that toxic world and it had nearly ended it all for me? I couldn't live with myself - with the embarrassment. I continued having panic attacks on and off for around 6 months, it was traumatising. It just shows you how powerful the mind is. I could run straight at 18 stone blokes, but now I was having irregular panic attacks, even when I was in the gym. I was just telling people I was a bit offside when I had one, but I still manged to keep going.

Then, a few months after in January 2017, another blow struck while I was at work. I got a phone call from the wife of my training partner to tell me he had died. I was still a mess in myself and now I had lost someone who was very important in my life. One of my best mates, what was going on? This brought me back down to earth and made me realise just how short life was. I needed to pull myself out of this mess. I put my focus back into work and gave it everything. I knew that putting 150% into my work was the one thing that I loved the most and it saved me.

I decided to see a friend of mine, a doctor, about the panic attacks and said I was feeling faint. A lot due to the long hours I was working. He came to the conclusion that I was exhausted and told me to have some glucose whenever I felt like this. I started to drink a Lucozade every day to combat this. It helped me feel better as carbs are great for numbing you and calming your anxiety, that's why most people turn to chocolate and sugar when they're anxious and comfort eat. This became my new source of escaping, not eating loads of rubbish, but eating too much food and having too much Lucozade. I also wasn't training regularly because I was feeling sorry for myself because of my training partner dying. I was getting a little bit better, but deep down I was still distraught about what I had done and comfort eating to forget about it. Luckily, I had still been doing really well at work, earning good money and decided to take up some counselling. Finally! I wish I had started that 5 years before as that one session a week was making me feel better. I was gradually beginning to feel like myself again and starting to figure out how the mind worked. However, I was still searching for answers in the wrong places. I took over the café at the gym, spending most of my savings because I was hoping this could be my main source of income and I wouldn't have to work extremely long hours anymore. This soon went under and was a bad decision. During this time, I decided to find the money to buy another business, one where I had bought my gym clothes from for many years. I found the money in the wrong way though through a couple of loans. I had checked out all of the accounts of the business and it looked like a good acquisition. Soon after buying it, I realised it wasn't what it was made out to be and I also discovered that I wasn't passionate about, nor good at selling clothes. The business soon started to struggle, and I had no money left. This caused me more problems in myself and in life. My dad tried to give me the kick up the backside I needed; I had hit rock bottom yet again but in a different way. I had finally started having counselling the previous year and it was helping me to not resort to dealing with these pressures in a dangerous way like I'd done before. It was helping me keep calm and start to understand how the mind worked. My counsellor was brilliant but working on your mind is the same as the body, it's an ever day job - you can't expect to do it once a week and it be enough. I had stopped drinking after 2016, but I needed to do more to really work on myself.

I tried anti-depressants again after trying them for a short while during the summer of 2014. However, they were making me sick every day. I was still playing rugby, so I stopped taking them. This time, I remember taking my first tablet one day and my youngest sister offering me some *"Calms"*, the natural anxiety remedy. This was a major turning point for me, it changed my life. I thought, *"what the hell am I doing taking one tablet to cure the anxiety from taking another tablet?"* What a stupid idea this is and what a horrible way to live. I was so annoyed with myself for getting into the state I found myself in and even considering taking anti-depressants. I mean I've nothing against people who do take them, everyone faces their challenges differently, but I know they do not get rid of the problem - they just numb you.

I used the pain and self-frustration to vow to myself never again was I going to let myself slide or feel sorry for myself. I was going to attack my problems like I was raised to do, no fear, no excuses, they were my problems. These problems were nobody else's fault and I needed to get a grip of myself, organise my thoughts and get back to living an amazing life, instead of wallowing in self-pity. I soon felt a hunger back for life that I hadn't had for a long time.

Around the same time, my mum gave me a book she had read years ago and told me it would help me out. It was Anthony Robbins *'Awaken the Giant Within'*. As soon as I started to read it, I became so excited because I realised everything that had happened was my own fault, but by changing the way I thought about things, I could change everything in my life. Since then, I have been completely obsessed with getting better every day and I now love my life again. I will go into more detail later in the book. I'm back to my best fitness wise and my anger has gone. I just love every day. All through understanding the power of my mind and how to use it and not let it destroy me and what to focus on. That's why I've written this book, to tell you everything I have learnt and hope that it can change your life and make your world a better place.

Too many of us have problems that we won't admit to. I remember one night at a party, when I was 18, an old friend of my dad's turned around to me and said that alcohol was the Devil and to avoid it. I wish I had listened to his advice; it would have saved me from so many problems.

So many of us have problems that are caused by drinking. Whether it's depending on it to relax, drinking too much at the weekend and it ruins the rest of the week, or binge drinking and doing stupid things that we'd never do without it like taking drugs, fighting, or abusing the people we love. We hide these problems because we are scared to face them as we are terrified to confront our demons.

I'm telling you from personal experience, we all have our demons but unless we face them, we are never going to be happy. We are always going to be living in fear of ourselves and only be one step away from pressing the self-destruct button like I did. On a positive note, if you want to find real happiness, it lies behind being honest with yourself, facing your demons and working on yourself. We all have bad things happen to us, we all have our demons, but the difference is, the people who go on to live an amazing life deal with their problems head on, take great confidence from it and feel unstoppable.

They take on the world in a positive way and I hope this book will motivate you to do the same.

Chapter 2
Life is always happening for you not to you

In life we are all going to have really bad things happen to us. We are all going to hit rock bottom and have to claw our way out of it and find ourselves again. This is one of life's big challenges, to realise that maybe life isn't being cruel to us in the hard times and that maybe it's just pushing us so that we can actually learn to improve ourselves and grow as people.

Take a moment to think to yourself. Have you had something happen to you which, at the time, you thought would be unbearable and you wouldn't be able to cope with? Then a few years down the line, you look back and think, *"I get why that happened to me and I'm probably glad it happened."* For example, not getting a promotion in work that you really wanted, but then finding a better job you prefer and being glad you didn't get that original promotion.

Could we all even go as far as saying things that, at the time seemed like the end of the world turned out to be the best things that happened to us? Whether it was splitting up with a boyfriend or girlfriend or losing your job. Could it be that these things pushed you down a different path to the point you were grateful? Personally, I am a big believer in fate - that life is already set out and all you can do is give it your best and try and be the best person you can possibly be. The rest is already going to happen and will take care of itself. I feel this is the best way to see life, keeping you strong and hopeful on the tougher days. My biggest example is my professional rugby league career, it had always been my dream to be a professional sportsman. I had dedicated my whole life to achieving that goal, but unfortunately for the reasons I explained at the start of this book, I messed it up for myself. I always dreaded and feared the thought of failing, the thought of letting myself down and the thought of having to go and get a proper job made me feel physically sick. It turned out to be one of the best things that happened to me. I mean it took me a long time to get over what happened in my life and during my career, but as I sit here writing this book today, I am so happy it didn't work out for me. Now I have a story that I can use to help anyone struggling in this life and show them how to find the most important thing in this world, self- happiness - which very few of us know how to master.

Most of us still think that self-happiness comes from how we look, how many likes/followers we get on social media or how much money we earn. Don't get me wrong money makes being happier easier but none of these are the answer. Don't we all want to feel good about ourselves? To feel good about yourself you need to find your inner purpose and what you were put on this earth to do. For me, I believe

I'm here to help as many people as possible change their mental and physical health. You could create an impact on people in a variety of different ways, whether it's teaching kids, helping out with charity work or being a nurse or doctor. Finding your purpose and a way of giving back to the world will find you the happiness you're after.

I now firmly believe that everything that happens to us in life is just part of a process to push us until we find out that this game is all a matter of perception. Any setbacks and problems just allow us to grow stronger and realise our lives are all within our own control. Our lives are in our own hands, but they are only in our own hands if we realise that our thoughts control our lives. If something doesn't work out and go right, we can't think the world is unfair we need to accept that it is time to step up. Life is telling us to work on ourselves, whether it's professionally or personally. No matter how convinced we are that we are on the right path - life knows better.

If we have this attitude that life is always happening for us, nothing can stop us from achieving the extraordinary life we were put on this earth to live. It's all down to you. Do you want to take the easy route and sit on the couch watching the news believing the world is a horrible place? Feeling sorry for yourself because of the pandemic and how hard it's been for you? Or do you want to take the positive approach? Spend more time working on yourself, take time to step back and find out what really makes you happy. Whether it's the simple things like a walk and a coffee with friends or realising how good exercising makes you feel and how it puts you in a better place for the day. Or using it as a time to do things you'd never normally have time to do. I have spent the time during this 2020/21 lockdown turning my life around, even though I've been in one of the hardest hit industries. Years ago, I would have felt sorry for myself and thought the world was against me, now my mentality means I see this sort of thing as a new challenge. I've used the time to read around 20 self- improvement books and complete a counselling and a life coaching course allowing me to step up and start working with people who are suicidal. I wanted to do this because I felt that low myself and bounced back. There is a way out. I now know that our mind is built to protect us in life, not to help us enjoy life. I've learnt that the mind is always working against you, not for you, if you don't learn to control your thoughts it can be a very destructive force.

One other important fact about life is that if you don't face and overcome a challenge the first time it's thrown at you, life will throw the same challenge at you again and again. Not because life is mean but because life wants us to be the best we can be. Life wants us to make a difference in the world. The world needs us all to be at our best and realise our full potential. Life doesn't need us to succumb to a lifetime of negativity and hate. Too many people have already done that, life needs us to grow from our challenges and mistakes, make the world a better place and in doing so see all the magic and beauty there is in this world.

So, whenever a challenge comes up in this life you need to realise it's a positive thing. It's a way to progress as a person and that's what happiness is. One of my favourite quotes on this topic I learnt from my hero Anthony Robbins, the guy whose book changed my life. When talking about how to live a happy life and encountering a problem he discusses that your attitude has got to be, *"I must tackle this problem now, immediately before anything else."* Give this a go the next time something arises that you're scared of facing, watch how it changes your life, I promise you this type of personal growth will give you a buzz of self-love and self-confidence that nothing else can give you.

I guarantee there will be some people who may struggle with this analogy of life happening for you, not to you. They'll probably think, "yeah, it's easy for you to say Joe" which I completely understand, but the people who survive these atrocities are the people who take what has happened to them in their lives and use it as an extremely powerful energy source to drive change in the world. They raise tremendous amounts of money to help fight cancer in children or they become inspirational speakers for peace in the world. The world needs these people although it must be horrendously hard to do. The people who experience these horrible things and don't take this attitude either let it ruin their lives or let their pain come out in negative ways. Which proves again, no matter what life throws at you, you will find the world really is an amazing place if you start to believe this.

We all want to be strong, independent people who can deal with anything. People who don't give into their fears and have the confidence to take on the world. How do we get this confidence and personal strength? Let's compare it to lifting weights in the gym, how do we get stronger muscles? We lift heavier weights and how do we get our muscles to adapt so that we find that weight easier? We keep practising those lifts and keep trying to improve the weight we lift or the reps we do. So, as simple as it sounds it's the same method for growing as a person in life. The bigger challenges we face and overcome, the bigger and stronger we're going to become as a person. We all want to be people who don't budge at the sign of a challenge. We all want to be people who can handle leading a family, who can handle being rich and having power or fame when we

achieve our goals. So how do we do this? By constantly facing our challenges, being positive and growing from them.
Otherwise, if we didn't face these things head on, we'd never handle them.

Let's use parenting as an example. If we were brought up and had no challenges and developed few life skills, would we make a good parent? Of course not, because when our child misbehaved or came home from school upset, we wouldn't have a clue how to do deal with it. So, all these problems we face aren't negative signs, they're just things we need to complete to be able to move on to that next stage in our lives. Another favourite quote of mine is, "your biggest problem is you think you shouldn't have any". We are always going to have problems in our lives, but it's about making them better problems.

To be honest we need problems in our lives otherwise we'd get so bored. Our lives would be too certain, and we'd lose the will to live. We need excitement and uncertainty to get us out of bed in the morning.

Some people avoid uncertainty and stay in the same old safe jobs all their life. They know that as long as they never put a foot wrong, they'll never get sacked. This is understandable with pressures like looking after your family, but because they never face their fears and try and grow, they never find out what they were meant to achieve in this world. To me, this is a waste of a life.

So just remember to flip a challenge on its head next time it comes along and don't go into self-pity mode. Think, "what's life trying to teach me here? How do I need to improve?" If you ever feel frustrated and think things aren't improving like you'd like them to - don't complain. Take action and go from feeling frustrated to energised in five minutes. This is what I do, and I usually find a new idea. Whether it's writing this book or doing live bootcamps on social media, I can't wait to take on the next challenge and improve again. If you want to be better at anything, life will throw you the opportunities to do so. These opportunities pop up every day, you've just got to take them positively. If you face them head on, make mistakes and learn from them, then so what? Don't be afraid to fail - your failures are what you grow from. Be clever enough to not make the same mistake twice and I promise you can become anyone you want to in this life.

Chapter 3
The mental and physical benefits of exercise and the right nutrition

When it comes to your diet, I recommend avoiding bad foods such as those high in sugar and takeaways apart from a once a week treat, depending on how healthy you are. Through the week I recommend sticking to eating balanced, regular meals making sure you eat breakfast and snack on the right types of foods. Eat a high protein, (red meat, fish, chicken, eggs and nuts), natural diet. Add carbohydrates into your meals as the day goes on or around training as too many can make you sluggish. Stick to good carbohydrate sources that are slow release in energy like brown rice, sweet potato and oats. Also, eat vegetables twice a day and have a few portions of fruit, but not too many. Don't go having 3-4 fruit smoothies a day as there are natural sugars in fruit, so too much won't do you any good.

For many of us, it isn't much of a secret that eating healthily and keeping fit makes us feel better, but to the people who struggle with this - I want to reinforce just how important it is.

The trouble with exercise for most people is that you must confront the fear of being in a gym or class environment before you can experience the benefits of it. There are plenty of people showing off their amazing figures in crop tops and stringer vests and when you're not happy with your own physical shape, it can be quite intimidating.

The benefits of facing these challenges and getting over this fear of exercising far outweigh the initial feeling of dread you might encounter the first time you enter a gym. If you've ever been to the gym and done some heavy weights or an intense circuit class, you'll have felt a high like no other. It will make you feel like a completely different person, full of confidence who can take on anything the world throws at you. It's amazing the difference just a one-hour session or a bootcamp class can have on your mood.

When you exercise and get your heart rate up, your brain releases endorphins which make you feel great and boost your energy levels.
The other things that have a similar effect are sex and dark chocolate - but dark chocolate isn't very good for you apart from maybe the odd piece, so exercise is the easiest and healthiest way to get this feeling in your life. So why wouldn't you want that feeling every day in life even if it takes just a few burpees to achieve it?

A lot of people go to the gym to look good and feel better in their own skin. Why do they want this? Mainly to feel good about themselves, but in some cases to help them find love. It is usually easier to get the attention of the type of people you're looking to find love with when you are in really good shape. I have trained a lot of people who have worked really hard on their fitness and then found love. We must remember that happiness on the inside is the key to happiness on the outside, so slacking off the gym and your diet is a dangerous path. No matter how good your life or relationship is. Firstly, because too many of us still don't realise the mental benefit of training. We have a mental health pandemic in this country which I know first-hand. Fitness could be part of the cure, but it is so overlooked.

Sometimes, when people encounter mental health problems, they've lost the ability to feel good about themself and their body. They've lost the confidence to overcome challenges and become a stronger person. They've lost the buzz of meeting similar, likeminded positive people and they think the world is full of negative individuals. So training is one of the biggest steps to changing your life. I would always tell people to focus on the mental benefits of training because it makes you feel good. People often discuss how many times a week you should train. I believe on the days you don't exercise; you don't feel as good and as mentally switched on - so why not train every day? Even if some days it's just a power walk or a lightweight session to get your body sweating. Then even have a shower and turn it cold for 30 seconds for a further natural hit of endorphins! Then you're set for the day and in a totally different place than if you didn't train. When you're tired and your body is aching like mad, go and do something steady like an arm session or a light jog to get your body loose and moving - you'll feel so much better.

We all have days where we don't feel like training, myself included even though it's my passion and my job. I know if I push myself to face it, I'll be a different person afterwards. Some days, I can roll up to the gym and my head is telling me, *"I can't do this today - I'm shattered."* Within an hour of a good session, I'm having a laugh with my training partner and we are pushing each other. I feel on top of the world again. I can't sit still, I have that much energy, which puts me in a much better mental state to go back to work and help my clients achieve their goals and feel better about themselves.

So many people miss out on all this fun and feeling good through their own fears. With their negative self-talk and excuses, *"I can't do this; I can't do that. I have no motivation."* These are just things we say to make ourselves feel better. I've trained people in their mid-80s who've have been extremely fit and others with only one arm that works. They don't make excuses.

I know it is hard if you've got a family and young kids, but some gyms are open 24/7 these days. Get up super early and try for 30 minutes and you'll be a totally different person for the rest of the day and more likely to be more productive and handle situations a lot better. You'll never feel fully happy in yourself giving yourself excuses. You will feel truly happy in yourself by putting yourself in places you feel uncomfortable, pushing through and coming out the other side of it laughing and joking with other members of the class. So, focus on the mental benefits over your physical body. Yes, you do have to look after your body, but most people worry too much about this - one slight ache and it's an easy way out for them not to do something. Remember this if your mind is right your body can withstand anything. Look at all the people who survived Auschwitz on barely any food each day in freezing temperatures without warm clothes. It was their mind that got them through that. If they can withstand detrimental physical conditions and still come out alive, I'm sure everyone can keep fit by doing some sort of exercise.

Even though it is very sad, one of my favourite stories of the power of the mind over body comes from the book '*Man's*

Search for Meaning' written by Auschwitz survivor, Viktor Frankl. He depicts the story of a fellow campmate who had a dream that they were going to be liberated on a certain date. He was full of excitement because he thought the date was coming. He had no problems with motivation to do the horrible jobs he had given to him because of this dream. The day came in which his dream said they were going to be liberated, nothing happened, and he died the next day. His mind gave up, so his body did too. It just shows how powerful the mind is and if you keep the mind healthy, the body will follow.

When it comes to training, I recommend doing all different types of exercise. Cardiovascular work which could be circuits, running or cycling. This will look after your heart and lungs to keep them working at their best. Weights or resistance training to look after your muscles and your bones to protect yourself from posture problems including aches and pains. Also stretching, Yoga or Pilates to increase blood flow and keep your muscles loose so they don't break when training. Furthermore, you must keep mixing up your training to keep it exciting. Don't let yourself get bored, join in different classes, do some dancing - just keep your body moving. Never sit down for too long. We are not built to be sat at a desk for 8 hours a day, but that's part of our world now so we need to make sure we get moving as often as we can for the rest of the day. Whenever you get chance in life, get out and move in the fresh air. A good balance of these types of exercise is the secret to physical success.

When it comes to nutrition, this is as just important as physical exercise for having an impact on our mental health. These days, it's harder than ever to avoid bad food. There are takeaways on every street corner, you can even get them delivered to your front door so that you don't have to get off the couch for them. This has led to an obesity crisis that kills thousands of people daily in this country.
As well as putting people in an early grave it has also ruined the time people spend on this earth because food makes us feel better for the short term. Good food will make us feel better long term and give us sustained energy whilst bad food gives us a short energy boost and then drops our energy, so we crave more bad food.

So many people have become addicted to sugar. They use it as their source of feeling better, their source of feeling sorry for themselves and they become addicted to it eating hundreds of grams a day and feeling like they need it. This is exactly what the food companies selling these products want because people will keep buying them - feeling like they can't live without them. Sugar is a source of carbohydrates and carbohydrates, especially sugar, can help to calm us down when we are feeling anxious.

Therefore, so many people put a lot of weight on when they are stressed. I know because I've done it myself. I wasn't eating lots of sugar, I was just eating too many meals to make myself feel better. It was still a bad habit and a hard habit to get out of because food is always going to be staring you in the face.

We tend to condone it to ourselves, *"it's ok we've eaten bad this week, but it's because the kids have been stressing me out. Work has been stressful; I've had no sleep; it's been everybody's birthday at work so there's been cake there every day."* As I said in the previous chapter, we are always going to have problems because they are there to help us grow. So, if we wait until we have no problems when it comes to sorting our diet out, we are never going to start, and you could waste your life being overweight, unhealthy and push yourself to an early grave. Why waste your life? Start now before you do anything else.

My personal advice for diet is to eat the foods that are natural - meat, fish, veg, fruit. It's simple, avoid anything processed. Enjoy a bad meal once a week. Life is for enjoying too, but most people struggle doing that and say, *"well if I'm too strict I'll fall of the rails"*, and by not being as strict they plan to eat one treat a day, get the taste for sugar and fall completely off the rails. So, the answer is simple but true again, be disciplined don't let those negative thoughts in and push yourself. You'll be surprised how good you'll feel about yourself for pushing yourself to be disciplined.

Also, you'll love how good you feel from eating regularly, snacking on the right foods and drinking two litres or more of water a day. You'll be more energetic, not need as much sleep, feel more confident about yourself and find it easier to make positive decisions. Studies have shown that just a 15% drop in hydration can lead to a significant lapse in concentration and performance. It just shows how important it is to stay hydrated and how bad you're likely to feel and function drinking diet coke all day.

Eating right and taking part in physical exercise is a big part of the battle of discovering how to be happy in yourself. By doing this, you'll have the foundations to start building the other blocks of a positive mind that I talk about in the other chapters of this book. There are a lot of positive people in a gym, but like I said – it's only half the battle. It's not good enough just going to the gym, if you're not going to work on yourself for the rest of the day and learn how to control your emotions. So, don't beat yourself up too much, there'll be people in the gym training like animals, but still a mess inside. You may have the rest of the mindset areas cracked that I talk about in this book and just need to work on your fitness and diet to complete yourself and start living your dream life. Although exercise and nutrition are half the battle to feeling great, it is just as important to work on the rest of the topics I talk about in this book. I was the prime example of this in my rugby days, physically tough but not as mentally strong as I needed to be for the challenge's life had to throw at me. I still see it a lot to this day. Many tough trainers, rugby players and fighters who train and play hard – you would think nothing would scare them. They can train, fight and play rugby all day but when it comes to being at home or dealing with emotions and situations in life, their weaknesses arise. Like I said, this is the honest view of myself before I started this path.

I personally think it's a lot harder to be tough in life than it is in the gym, on the field or in the ring. So many people / athletes have alcohol problems because they haven't got a positive escape method. They can't deal with their emotions or demons as well when they're not doing what they love. Some of them live very unhappy lives away from the gym or their sport. It was my downfall and I want to help as many people as I can to make sure it's not their ruin too. It's just hard to be that honest with yourself and not play down your problems.

The goal is to be fit, not just physically fit - to be truly happy you must be emotionally sound too.

Chapter 4
Habits

Habits are the main thing that separates a successful life from an unsuccessful one. Successful people love to talk about their habits and how they have led them to success, while unsuccessful people try to avoid talking about theirs, usually because it's what's holding them back in life.

Negative habits even in the simplest form may not seem like the end of the world at the time, but it's the effect they have on our day to day lives that we brush over too much. Whether it's a couple of drinks daily, or £50.00 a week on cigarettes, these negative habits are usually there to make us feel better, to relieve our pain and enhance our pleasure for a short time. The truth is, these usually cause more pain in the future and we can become addicted to them without even knowing. We become dependent and condone them. We might say, *"it's only one glass per night and it could be worse."* We compare ourselves to people who are doing worse. Surely, you'd feel much happier in yourself by telling people your positive habits and how well your life's going?

The truth is, we are scared of these positive habits because they mean confronting our fears, insecurities and even standing up to our friends who may be bad influences on us.

They may think were boring if we don't drink as much or don't go out for a cig break with them at work. Do you really want to be like this? Those friends aren't really friends - they just drag you into their habits to make themselves feel better.

Negative habits are easy to slip into, but very hard to get out of. The longer you've been participating in negative habits, the longer it's going to take you to get out of them. You become addicted to them, they become your source of comfort and whenever something goes wrong, you go back to them. These negative habits usually come from the fear that we're not good enough, that we might try and fail, that people may judge us if we do something positive to break our patterns and leave them behind. Then you stay with these problems and use them as an excuse to delay dealing with them. It's so common for me to hear people make excuses to change in the future but not immediately.

Let me tell you a hard home truth, if you wait for the right time, it's never going to come because you're always going to have problems and challenges. Things you can use as an excuse. If you find excuses, you're never going to start. Before you know it another 10 years will have gone by, you'll be a couple more stone overweight and starting to worry about cancer taking your life early because you've smoked for that long.

So how to you break a bad habit?
You must first obviously be honest with yourself that you need to break it and identify what pleasure you link to the bad habit. For example, calming your anxiety or removing stress from your work. Then, you need to sit down and write out all the pain this bad habit could bring you. Using smoking as an example, you could write down the life experiences you could miss out on. You really need to scare yourself with this, the more pain you can associate with the habit, the easier it will be to stop. Then you have to write down all the positive things that could happen if you stopped smoking and make them as exciting as possible. For example, having an extra £200 a month to spend, living to see your grandchildren, looking better in yourself and having more self-confidence. Make it as exciting as possible and think of as many reasons as you can.

Another big tip is changing your environment. When you've had a bad habit for so long, you have trained your subconscious mind to do something without even letting the conscious mind come in and stop you. Start by removing any signs of your bad habit from your life. Don't keep them there and rely on your willpower, because that means you're probably still thinking about going back to them. It

will be hard, but you must avoid being near anyone who smokes for a while - even if they're your
best friends. To break the habit will be tough, but it's your life remember and just think about all the pain it's going to cause you if you don't change this bad habit.

Being with a friend who is smoking while you're trying to break the pattern will be a nightmare. They'll start feeling bad about themselves for not trying to break the habit and offer you one to make themselves feel better.

Some of you might be thinking, *"but they're my friends - they wouldn't do that to me"* but trust me you wouldn't believe how many of our actions come from how we feel about ourselves. People will go to great lengths to feel good about themself and stay away from facing their own fears, even if they are the nicest person in the world. To change a habit, we need to make the habit invisible.
So, to change a negative habit firstly we need to associate as much pain as possible with it. Secondly, we need to associate as much pleasure as possible with stopping the habit. Then we need to change the environment, so the habit is invisible. Finally, we need to replace the habit with a positive habit.

Why don't we have a look at another bad habit like having a drink before you going to bed at night to relax you, what could you do to replace this habit?

You could join the gym and do an exercise class where you let all your stresses out from your day in a positive manner. Trust me you'll struggle to stay awake after a busy day at work followed by a heart raising bootcamp class. You could go for a walk with a friend in the fresh air. This will really help you clear your head and get you into a positive mindset.

What difference do positive habits make to your life? Positive habits make you feel good. They give you momentum to attack the day like nothing else will. One positive habit will lead to the next and so on.

Positive habits will lead to a positive life, they will bring positive people into your life and more positive situations. For example, being positive and starting the gym will lead to you meeting new people and gaining more self- confidence. Starting your own business will lead to you meeting like-minded driven people who you will rub off on you. They will bring more positivity and energy into your life.

Positive habits will lead to more self-confidence. This confidence is real confidence, not the confidence you get after a drink because you don't care what anyone says. This is real self-built confidence that takes hard work to build, but that hard work gives you so much strength that you feel unbreakable.

Good habits also lead to everything else that's already in your life working better, for example going to the gym and keeping fit will lead to you having more energy and excitement in your relationships. Also, going into the self-improvement mode and discovering your own strengths and weaknesses will allow you to take more appropriate action when your partner is having a bad day. You will be able to find solutions in an argument, rather than exploding at your partner. With this positive approach your relationship will flourish.

How much your life can change by replacing your bad habits for more positive ones is unlimited. You'll be shocked at how quickly a few good habits can completely change the course of your life.

18 months ago, at the start of my journey, I implemented a great little habit to start my day. I read about it in the Anthony Robbins book I have mentioned previously. Every morning after having my breakfast, coffee and taking the dog for a walk, I sit down and put some positive music on. I then do 20 shoulder presses as fast as I can for two rounds with a slight pause in between sets. Then another round of

ten shoulder presses. Whilst doing this, I breath in on the downward phase of the movement and breath out as I press my arms up. This is to get your blood flowing; get you awake and get your mind in a positive state. I then spend a few minutes thinking of three things I'm truly grateful for. One minute on each one and I truly step into the moment no matter how simple it is. I really feel like I'm experiencing that situation or feeling again. I personally choose my dog, my family and my friends as my three every day but you can choose whatever you like. Next, I spend a minute imagining something healing in my life, so any current little problem going on such as the gyms being shut during lockdown. I step into the moment of teaching my first class back and how good it will feel. For the last three minutes, I think of three things I want to achieve and visualise them as strongly as possible. Visualisation is such a powerful tool, as our mind doesn't know the difference between us imagining something and it actually happening in our lives.

I do this morning routine seven days a week without fail. It normally takes me 10 minutes, but sometimes I enjoy it that much I get carried away and go for longer. If you feel like you haven't got time in the morning, guess what, get up earlier and this habit will make you feel amazing for the rest of the day. It stops you from feeling down or angry because you're too busy feeling grateful for what you have in life and excited for achieving your future dreams. Give it a go - you won't regret it.

Don't overthink getting better with your habits. Don't expect to go from being a smoker to being as fit as everyone else in the gym in two weeks. Focus on trying as hard as you can, being the best that you can be and just improving 1% at everything you do every day. This isn't hard to do and if you improve 1% at everything you do each day over the year, you'll be 365% better! Just imagine how much that will change your life!

What are some other good habits that will improve your life?
The obvious ones we've already spoken about. Exercising, eating the right foods and getting outside on a daily basis. We all spend way too long sat inside, especially in the winter and our bodies are not built for being sat down. Our respiratory systems weren't built for breathing heating and air conditioning in all day. No wonder we feel stressed, it's because our bodies are strained from all the rubbish, we're breathing in. Another great habit to have is helping people, whether that's giving the homeless man outside the shop his dinner every day or helping raise money for a charity, I guarantee you will feel ten times as good for doing this compared to buying yourself a new car or a McDonalds.

We were all put on this earth to be exceptional human beings and we all have that power to change the world in our own way, it's just whether we realise how much a difference our little actions every day can make to the world. Other good habits to maintain are things like *"to do lists"* at work. It is very important be early to work then you're not late and stressed and starting off on the wrong foot.

Keep your desk or your house clean, make your bed every day. Simple little things to do will make you feel so much better. Positivity and little efforts will help stop negativity coming into your day. You're never going to have a positive day if you wake up five minutes before work resulting in you being late. Your day is already ruined if you do that, but so many of us still do this and self- sabotage on a daily basis. What a shame when we have all got so much to give to this world.

Get up earlier, if you're tired go to bed earlier. We all like a bit of TV and a sit down at night but we don't need to watch three hours of a series every night. Life is too short to ruin your day just so you can find out who the murderer is on your favourite drama. That will still be there with your cup of tea the next night.

Practise the morning routine I talked to you about or just write down three things you're grateful for every morning. Get into work early and say hello to as many people as you can. Take the time to ask them how they are doing. You never know how a small act of kindness will pay you back in the future. I'm a big believer in that karma works both ways and when you are nice to people, life will pay you back - sometimes in indirect ways that you would never expect. That's why even in the time I've struggled financially, I've still given a small amount of money to charity every month.

When you're in work be positive, be productive and you never know where that will get you. Maybe a promotion? More money, a day off as a thank you and a present at Christmas? All these small positive habits will lead to all sorts of positive outcomes that will change your life and perspective of the world. As much as a good diet gives us energy and quality sleep, I believe energy also comes from making yourself an exciting life and good habits. For example, when you get up at 3am to go on holiday - the lack of sleep never bothers you then, so why not live a life that excites you that much and you'll never have to worry about lack of sleep again? Good habits will change your life - just one habit at a time.

Chapter 5
Beliefs

Beliefs are what shape our lives, whether it's our beliefs about the world or our beliefs about ourselves. Our beliefs decide whether we feel good about ourselves and good about the world, or bad about ourselves and like the world is against us.

Like I've said in previous chapters, the world is never against us. No matter what happens to us, life throws us challenges to make sure we are constantly growing. The world wants to push us in the right direction.

Nevertheless, very few people have the strength to have that positive empowering belief. Most of us have so many negative beliefs that they take over our lives and stop us from fulfilling our potential. For example, many of us believe that our lives depend on politicians and governments. This belief has never been shown more strongly than when *"Brexit"* happened in this country and there were hundreds of kids stood outside parliament with banners saying, *"Brexit has ruined my future."* Whatever your belief on this, I'm personally not really into politics but when I saw this I thought, *"what a horrible limiting belief to have."* To be fair, it's more of an excuse really to make yourself feel better, *"I can't succeed because of Brexit. I can't succeed because Boris has locked us down. I can't succeed because I didn't have money growing up and had a hard upbringing"*, are some of the most common limiting beliefs that I hear. These are life destroying and complete excuses.

If people can rise from poverty to be millionaires, if people can come out of Auschwitz and use their story to change the world like Viktor Frankl, if the 3 richest people in the world can come close to doubling their net worth during the pandemic - is there really any excuse? No matter what's going on in the world, can you really let your limiting beliefs ruin your life and blame other people or circumstances for your failures?

No! There is never an excuse. You are only ever competing against yourself in this life. Competing against your limiting beliefs and how productive, resourceful and creative you can be. If there are tougher financial circumstances around at the time, this only means one thing - you have to be more resourceful. The main excuse for failing usually comes from a negative belief system about a lack of resources. For example, a lack of money and it's never usually a lack of resources that is the problem, it's more about a lack of resourcefulness - which is you not using your skills to the best of your ability. So, your resources could be your skillset such as being good at writing, selling things, dealing with people or online marketing. Or resources could be something that you own that could bring you money in like if you have a big van, you could go and earn money doing home removals. We all have resources, whether it's skills we have or things we own that could increase our income. We usually aren't resourceful enough to use them to bring us more money in.

In this media obsessed world that we live in, it's so easy to think the world's a horrible place. This is because the media always focusses on negativity because it sells better and grabs attention. This leads to us having negative, limiting beliefs about the world. We think the world is in a terrible place. Everyone's trying to fight and kill each other and there's a virus taking over the world. Are we ever going to get back to normal? All super limiting beliefs that can destroy your life. Many people live off this negative news we're fed and let it shape their lives - which is a travesty in my opinion.

To change your beliefs on the world, I advise you strongly to stay away from the news. Stay away from negative people who constantly moan about the world. Get outside and look at the amazing things being done every day. Go and work in a food bank for a day or help with a local charity. Take part in a 5k or 10k run/walk and see all the people pushing their bodies to raise money for all sorts of causes and make a difference in the world.

Looking at our own beliefs is so important. Let's say you have a goal you want to achieve - like finding the perfect partner. Your inner beliefs tell you that there isn't a perfect partner out there for you, so because of this you will more than likely take lousy action to achieve this goal. You might meet up with someone and because your beliefs are so negative about men/women and love, you don't show much enthusiasm and positivity in your conversation. Your date doesn't go well, and the person decides not to go on another date with you. This reinforces your negative limiting belief that there isn't a perfect partner out there for you.

But then again, let's say you have a positive empowering belief that you are 100% sure that the right partner is waiting out there for you in your life. When your date comes along, you'll be full of optimism and positivity and you'll dress your best, you'll use your best perfume/aftershave, you'll walk into the date with positivity and excitement. You'll be full of conversation and it will rub off on your date and you'll have a great night. Then, your date will be more likely to go out again with you, reinforcing your positive beliefs about finding the right partner. See how important your beliefs are?

Without positive beliefs you've no chance of achieving your goals no matter how hard you try. To achieve anything in this life, you really need to believe you can do it and have some strong positive empowering beliefs about yourself and your own personal strengths. Yes, we all have our doubts even the most successful people in the world have their self-doubts, but we must have some strong beliefs about ourselves to override them and make sure our life is successful.

I think beliefs are hugely important in the world of sport. For example, when it comes to winning titles and trophies, it's usually teams who believe in themselves the most who get over the line first. So, when they have a bad day or lose a game, they still believe that they are the best and bounce back stronger. On the other hand, teams with less positive beliefs find negatives about themselves and their teammates. When things start to go wrong, they are more likely to go on a downward spiral when they start losing a few games.

Let's take the late great Muhammad Ali, for example, he was known for what we call *"Affirmations"* about himself. He would constantly tell everyone he was the best of all time and by doing this he showed his belief in himself and made the whole world believe the same. To be successful you must be ultra-confident in yourself and have as many empowering beliefs as possible. Your head has to be held up all the time, your shoulders back, you need to think and act with confidence and believe that you are going to achieve your goals. Walking around looking at the floor with your shoulders hunched and a set of negative beliefs about yourself, no matter how hard you try, isn't going to achieve anything.

Most of the people who have achieved amazing things in this life, that no one outside of themselves believed they could, did this because their beliefs were so strong. For example, people in England laughed at *Arnold Schwarzenegger* when he was over here starting his bodybuilding training and he told everyone he was going to be the greatest of all time and conquer Hollywood.

Everyone training in the same gym as him at the time laughed at him and just look what he achieved. The people who made the first light bulb, the first smartphone, were all laughed at before they achieved their goal. What got them over the line? Their beliefs! When you believe something so strongly, anything is possible because you'll keep going and going until you achieve your goal. No matter how many times you fail, your beliefs will keep pulling you over the line.

How many times have you heard the saying, *"don't judge a book by its cover?"* What does this mean? It means we can all be guilty of looking at someone and having a set of beliefs about the way they are and what sort of person they'll be just from the way they look. I am sure it's quite easy to do the same with myself with the tattoos that I have on my hands and arms. This usually fills us full of negative beliefs about a person and ruins the great opportunity of getting to know them and finding out what they're really like. We usually get annoyed with someone over a certain situation when we don't even know them. For example, being annoyed with a particular point of view on politics or any situation in the world that we hear on the TV or on social media that goes against your beliefs. You could immediately make all sorts of assumptions about them, they're selfish, they're higher class, they don't know what it's like to work for a living.

Suddenly, you don't like someone you've never met. When if you actually broke past these limiting beliefs and looked into the person or got to know them, you'd possibly find they've had a really challenging life and had some horrible things happen to them. They could actually be a really a nice person. We all spend most of the time seeing the world through our own eyes, seeing our problems as the worst ones in the world. If we can break past these limiting beliefs by trying our best to think positively about a person first, we can change our own world and make it a much happier place.

By having the positive belief that people are just making their decisions based on their own world and experiences, this will change your life and you'll spend so much less time getting frustrated with people and actually enjoy their company. This will allow you to meet more people who may make a massive difference in your life and spend more of your day in a positive state.

So, how do we create some positive beliefs about ourselves if we need to get rid of our negative beliefs first? Say the belief that you wanted to change is that you believe you are not very good at operating computers and it was holding you back from the jobs you wanted in life. Firstly, you would take up a computer course that helped you become better on a computer. Secondly, you would change your belief from, *"I'm not very good on computers"*, to, *"I am working hard and improving on computers."* By improving your self-talk, your mind starts to believe what it hears when you're saying these new positive beliefs and stops you from limiting yourself. Then, every time you learn something new or do something better on the computer, you would have more things to back up your new belief and continue to improve moving forward. This method can be used for anything whether it's computers, sports or going to the gym. By changing your beliefs, self–talk and taking action to improve a skill, you can change anything in your life by making your beliefs empowering ones.

Chapter 6
How to deal with people

Dealing with people is such a massive part of our lives but yet so many of us fail to master it. Our relationships with people define how successful and happy we are in life and to do this we must have good relationships with people that bring us happiness and in turn can bring us success. To have good relationships with people, we must understand how to deal with people and understand them especially when they are having a bad day.

We spend so much of our time messing up our lives by judging people and falling out with them. We make it so much harder for ourselves to be happy and successful.

Everyone knows somebody successful and usually what is it that stands out most about them? They have a way of dealing with people, a way of coming across as successful and intelligent. They have a way of persuading you that their product is the best or that they're the person you want to hire for their service. Good salespeople are great communicators. They know how to step into your world, find out what your greatest needs are, what your greatest areas of pain are and what you really want in life. To be successful in life we all need to become great salespeople.

We need to be able to step into the shoes of other people, listen to them, understand their desires and opinions on things and not just talk about ourselves and put our point across to make ourselves feel better.

One of the best pieces of advice I can give you about dealing with people is to be a good listener. Why do we get on well with our best friends? For the reason that we think they're cool or because we think they'll spend lots of money on us on our birthdays? No not at all. It's simple, it's because they listen to our problems, step into our world, take our corner in every problem that we face and make us feel better about ourselves. So, to get on with people and be successful with dealing with them, we have got to be a friend to everyone we meet - it's that simple. We have got to build up a strong rapport with people. I know not everyone you meet will have the same interests as you, but I would suggest trying to find some common ground with the person you are talking to even if you don't have any - so that you can get along and either make them a friend or a business associate. The more people who like you and think you care about them, the more success you'll have in life in general.

Here is another big thing to think about, people like to talk about themselves. They like to talk about their own achievements and their own problems because it makes them feel better. Yes, our best friends will talk about us and try and help us out but if we want to build relationships with people who we are not as close with or don't really know, we have got to learn to listen to them and make them feel like they're the most important thing in the world. If you can learn to do this, then you'll never fail to make a connection with someone again. You'll always be able to get on with people from every walk of life and you'll have a very successful life in doing so.

A lot of the time, the things we struggle with most in our lives are conflicts with people. We tell them what we are not happy about, things they've done or the way they've acted. We make them feel bad so that they send the attack straight back at us and before we know it, *"World War 3"* has broken out. So, my biggest tip on this is to avoid arguing at all costs. Don't get me wrong, this is very challenging, and I struggle with it myself definitely, but if you can learn to get your point of view across without seeming offensive and causing an argument, then you'll be unstoppable. You'll be able to overcome every personal or work relationship challenge you have.

A great tip for when you need to raise a point of concern with someone, whether it is a family member or colleague is to deliver a positive point or compliment to them first. Tell them something they are good at or have done well in the past. Do this to show them that you care and you believe in them. For example, if you are bringing up a concern with a member of staff over a piece of work they've done, don't go in ripping their work to pieces.

Firstly, go in and complement the good stuff they do and how much you think of them and then tell them what you'd like them to do better or what they've done wrong. When it comes to your children for instance, tell them how proud of them you are for cleaning their bedroom last week before telling them off for not cleaning it this week.

Another good tactic for avoiding arguments is bringing the problem up indirectly. So, if a colleague has sent a piece of work over without enough detail in, you could go to them and say for example, *"I think you forgot to save your work. I don't think all of it has come across to me"*, and show them what you have received, which will probably lead the member of staff to realise they haven't gone into enough detail and they'll go back to work without you making them feel bad about themselves and starting an argument.

Often in life our insecurities and fears blow up if someone treats us badly. In these times although it's very hard, we need to understand that someone treating us badly is more to do with how they feel about themselves, rather than how they feel about us. Think of the happiest person that you know. Do they usually treat other people badly? Do they usually get into a lot of arguments? No, because they are happy on the inside, they don't need to shoot anyone down to make themselves feel better. They have less of their own insecurities, so little things don't bother them as much. People being successful doesn't bother this kind of people because they are facing their own fears and being positive about their own life, so they'll never get jealous or insecure over things. How many times have you seen a person try and shoot somebody down when they've done well? Why does this happen? It is because success causes great jealousy in people, it makes people wish that they could do the same and hate themselves for not having the strength to face their own fears. We have all had this happen to us in our lives and it can push us into the negative circle of feeling sorry for ourselves and holding resentment and anger towards people, and anger is a deadly emotion. It can destroy us. It nearly destroyed my life and I know I won't be the only person who can say that. So, how do we stop ourselves from feeling angry about how someone treats us? What someone does to us no matter how bad it is, whether it's hitting us, cheating on us or just calling us names, we need to realise that their actions have nothing to do with us and it's more how they feel about themselves. They are obviously very unhappy in their lives or dealing with something that's hurting them or there are things in their lives that have left them with mental scars that they haven't had the strength to face. This doesn't mean we can't be strong with people and tell them when they are out of line. We need to be strong with people so that they realise their mistakes and can grow as people. We just need to learn how to deal with it ourselves so that we don't take it to heart and it doesn't scar us.

Another massive step in self-improvement that helps us get on with people is acknowledging our own mistakes. For example, when we're having an argument with our partner, acknowledging the mistakes we've made with them first will make them feel better, help to build trust and help them to find it is easier to take your feelings into account. If you're not happy with them about something, because you've admitted your mistakes first, you're showing great honesty and strength. Or if it's with your staff when you're pointing out some mistakes they've made, tell them about previous mistakes you've made in the past and what you've learned from them. It will help you gain greater respect from your staff and build up their motivation. When they see that you too were once making mistakes like them and you still managed to be successful - it will also help create a good, honest working relationship where you can both laugh at previous mistakes and learn from them together.

Furthermore, another great but simple way to improve your relationships with people is to just make them feel important in your life. For example, texting your friends weekly, asking how they are and just talking about their lives, making them feel like they are important. This will help you build some great friendships where you'll find people will do anything in return for you because you made them feel special. If you can make someone feel important, they'll never feel alone and feel so good about themselves.

Also, an example in the workplace would be if you as the boss could take the time to ask each member of your staff how their family is and if there's anything you can do for them. This will produce so much enthusiasm for work because they love working for you and you'll get better results than you could have ever imagined. People just want to feel important and significant and even more so, they want to feel important in their work and friendship groups. It makes them feel special and wanted. It can work wonders for your life and for theirs with just a little bit of effort to make them feel that way.

Using encouragement to motivate people and holding them to positive high standards are other great ways to form great relationships and get the best out of them. People love to be encouraged - we all struggle for motivation at times so that little bit effort to motivate someone can go a long way to making someone feel like they are needed and appreciated in the workplace. Also, when trying to get the best out of somebody if they've done something that you're not happy with - hold them to a high standard. For example, if someone does a piece of work that's only half the quality you want from them, tell them it's not up to their usual very high standard and remind them of the exceptional work they have done previously, because that's how good they really are. People hate letting themselves down but love it when people believe in them and make them out to be something special because we all want to be very good at something and feel like we're clever or talented. When they know they can do better it motivates them to hit that high standard again because it gives them that belief that that's the standard they are, that they are a top-class worker because you believe they are. That's all the motivation they'll need to get it fixed because people hate dropping their standards - especially when someone has complimented them and told them they're good at something. This is a better way of motivating people than attacking them and making them feel worthless because by doing this, they then feel bad about themselves and hate you and have no motivation to complete the task you've asked of them to a high standard. So be clever with people, lift them up to motivate them and get the best out of them, don't drag them down.

Chapter 7
How to achieve anything you want to

Can you achieve anything you want to in this life? Can you achieve your dreams? Can anyone be a millionaire?

These are the big questions that most people spend their days doubting. Thinking that it's not possible, using all their negative beliefs to find the easy way out and prove that it's not true and that their circumstances or problems exempt them from having the life of their dreams.

I can tell you now, this is complete rubbish and a waste of the precious gift that is life. You can achieve everything you want to in life, but there are one or two deciding factors on how you go about achieving your dream life and the main one is using your god given gifts. I don't care who you are or what state your life's in right now, you have been given some gifts that you are amazing at whether it's playing sport, dealing with people or making peoples hair look nice. We have all been given something we're good at that can make us a millionaire, we just have to do enough of our work or work our way up in this area. For example, if you're a hairdresser - owning enough salons to make you a millionaire. If you're a doctor or nurse - working your way up to the top of the NHS or having your own private patients to earn more money to earn the life of our dreams.

It's that simple, so let's use my own example. To be a millionaire I would need to do around 28000 PT sessions a year or around 2300 a month, so there's obviously not enough time for that. Instead, I would need 15-20 personal trainers working under me who I coach, get clients for and take a cut. I would need my own gym on top of that to make up the money from memberships and classes. Enough to make myself a millionaire from my gift and my business. Yes, it is tough, but it doesn't take a genius to do this. So, to become a millionaire and have that dream life, you just need to be producing your god given talents enough times a week/month/year to create that money.

A lot of people spend too long chasing their dreams using things they're not good at or not physically built for. For example, if you're 5ft 2, being a world class basketball player is going to be extra difficult. You will have a lot of other gifts that you will find come naturally. You can use these to achieve anything you want from. That's my first tip to achieve what you want in life; you have to do something you're really good at. We are really good at something, so we just have to find that.

Secondly, you must change your physical and emotional

state before you can plan out how you're going to achieve your goal. Get out of the state of feeling sorry for yourself and get up. Get your body moving, do some exercise and get yourself feeling good. It is hard to write out some exciting action steps towards your goals when you're half asleep on the couch or watching something negative on the news. Taking part in physical exercise increases the feel-good hormone dopamine and decreases the stress hormone cortisol. So, if you plan your action steps towards your goals after exercising, you're a lot more likely to plan some positive, fearless actions steps that will increase your chance of success. Also spend some time thinking about the times you've done the best in your life when you've achieved or done the things, you're the proudest of.

This will get you feeling determined and confident in yourself because you're focussing on your own strengths and not your doubts and fears. Because again if you're in a negative emotional state, you're going to make some lousy decisions and create some poor action steps. They won't work, leading to you again reinforcing your limiting beliefs that you can't do this.

Thirdly you must, as mentioned in previous chapters, change your mindset because if you have negative beliefs about yourself or your goal, all the effort in the world isn't going to get you to it. So, you must write down a set of positive beliefs about yourself that are goal related because if you have negative beliefs, you'll try something without really believing you can achieve it. If the belief is not there, the best action in the world won't achieve your goals. It won't work and then you'll convince yourself you were right about being useless.

Furthermore, you must take massive action not just baby steps. Don't hold back and take small steps. Completely pack in smoking, apply for that new job or join the gym and book your first PT session all in the same night! Take it NOW, not next week, not tomorrow, not when the kids are behaving, not when you feel better or when you've spent a week on google searching for the best personal trainer. Do it now before you do anything else because if you put off doing it, you're giving yourself more chance of never taking that action.

So, if your goal is to run a marathon, just get out that door and run until you have to stop. Do the same the next day and the next and whilst you're doing this you can look for the best methods and best trainers, but all these things don't matter if you aren't out there every day grafting your socks off. So just go and do it now. So many people spend too long overthinking their goal and asking too many questions about what the way to do it is and miss out on the main part of achieving a goal. Just get started and start working hard! If you want a new job, apply for as many new jobs as possible in the next hour after reading this book. Hesitation kills momentum and momentum is what we need in life. It makes us feel like we're going places and makes us feel good. The bigger the action we take, the quicker we're going to get to our goals and the quicker you're going to feel like you've broken free from the shackles of fear that have been holding you back for so long.

Another amazing tip to achieve your goals would be to model someone who's already achieved it. It's so easy to model someone these days, literally every successful person in the world has either written a book or done a podcast/documentary on how they achieved their goals. All you have to do is go out and do exactly what they've done, copy their habits, take some of their actions and back it up with some of your new positive beliefs of your own.

For example, a lot of young lads want to be footballers and look up to Cristiano Ronaldo as being the best in the world. Well, his habits are no secret, everyone knows that he's the first one to training and the last one to leave. He works on his physical body more than most footballers and takes ice baths all night after a game to aid his recovery. So, you want to be the best footballer in the world?

Go and copy him! You just need the same work ethic! Basically, what he does is just work harder than everyone else - go and do the same!

Dwayne Johnson, Hollywood's highest paid actor - everyone knows he gets up at 4am and trains before most people are awake to get himself in the best emotional and physical state for the day. Then he goes to the movie set. You want to emulate his success? Go and copy him! For another example, studies showed that before Serena and Venus Williams hit the top of their sport, they had played and practised 10,000 hours of tennis! Want to emulate their success? Go play and practise as much as possible.

Is it me or are the rules to success really simple? They just take a lot of discipline and hard work?

To set out your goals the best way you can, you need to be precise with them. You need to write them down so you're being more honest about them and getting exactly what you want. Don't just say, *"I want more money",* because you might get a 50p a week pay rise as you weren't precise enough so say something like, *"earn an extra £50,000 a year by the end of 2021."* Your brain works better with precision and if you give it the outcome you want, it will find the best and quickest way possible to get you to that outcome. Even telling a friend will help because it will put a little bit of pressure on you to achieve it and bring with it extra self-motivation to achieve the goal. Or even better, hire someone who has achieved your goals before or who can help you achieve them. This will be so beneficial as they will increase your motivation, making it simpler for you to achieve by showing you the best techniques and the quickest ways to reach it. They will keep you on track on the days you feel like giving up. All successful people have good mentors or coaches they can turn to, to keep them on the right path. Every success comes from a coach bringing out the best in the team or an individual - nobody does it by themselves. So, it's very important you pick a great coach or mentor.

Another big question you'll get when it comes to goals is what happens if this approach doesn't work? Well guess what, it's a really simple answer again - try another way or another idea! Then if that doesn't work, try something else. Just keep trying until it works and you'll get over the line. It doesn't matter how many different things you have to try as long as you succeed does it? Most of the people who have had the greatest successes in this world have had the most number of setbacks, but they just kept going and learnt from their mistakes and tried different ways. Not many people get it right the first time, so don't be put off if your first idea or business plan doesn't get you the success you want - just keep going!

To help increase your motivation and increase the chances of succeeding, it's a good idea to write down the pain and pleasure linked with your goal. So, write down all the pain that not achieving or not trying to achieve your goal will cause. Make it as painful as possible to not take action and try everything to achieve your goals. Then write down all the ways you'll find pleasure in your life by achieving your goals.

The more pain you can link to staying where you are and the more pleasure you can attach to achieving your goals, the greater the chance you'll take better action and this will actually increase the chances of achieving your goals. By associating as much pleasure as possible, it will give you more reasons to keep going on the challenging days and when you encounter failure. Pain is also a great motivator, so the pain of staying where you are can be a great source of motivation to spur you on to keep fighting for your goals whatever it takes to reach them.

So, here's the full guide again:

1- Get yourself in the best state possible.

2- Change your beliefs.

3- Take massive action right now.

4- Write things down and be precise.

5- Model someone who has already achieved your goal.

6- Get a coach or friend to help you who has already achieved it.

7- Keep trying different methods until you get the winning formula.

Get started! Take action now! No excuses!

Chapter 8
It all starts with you

The simple answer to finding happiness, success and freeing yourself from your past troubles is the realisation that it all starts and ends with you. It's nobody else's fault. Yes, people can challenge you like mad and do horrible things to you at times but in the end it's all down to you, your beliefs and habits. It's all about the way you react to things and whether you can take the idea of life happening for you, not to you so that you take every setback or failure as an opportunity.

The attitude of, *"it all comes down to you"*, is one which I think makes life a lot easier and simpler. You don't have to worry about what other people are doing, how well they're doing or what they're doing to stop you succeeding because it doesn't matter. People use these things as an excuse not to achieve their goals, when really, they are just challenges life has asked you to face to motivate you to force you to grow and to push you in the right direction.

The main thing the top earners and happiest people put their success down to is self-improvement. Self-improvement looks different for lots of people, for some it's getting up at 4am to train – and for others it's cutting down on their drinking. Which is all fine, it's all about just moving in the right direction. It's about feeling like you're becoming a better person every day and being excited waking up every morning. That's happiness, not achieving a following on Instagram or not being wealthy and having a wealthy boyfriend/girlfriend who gives you a life where you don't have to work as much.

This road to happiness all comes from working on your progress as a person. This is what really equals happiness and self-improvement routines are what set us up for the day. They get us in a good mental state to attack the challenges life throws at us, keep us in a positive mindset and if we spend our time in this headspace – every day will be a good day because we decided it will be.

Some popular self-improvement techniques are:
- Getting up before sunrise.
- Meditation.
- Visualisation.
- Journaling or gratitude journaling.
- Ice baths.
- Religion/praying.
- Fitness/training.
- Doing challenges that make you face your fears (skydiving, firewalking).

I fully recommend you give all these a go, they all get your day off to a good start or give you a buzz like no other. Getting up before sunrise will show to you that the negative voice in your mind has no power over you. Sky diving or fire walking can show you that if you push through your fears, you can achieve anything and get a high that nothing else will give you. Meditation will help bring peace to your thoughts and not let your mind run riot over any slight problem.

If you want to improve yourself the most, I recommend incorporating all of these ideas into your life.
Religion is one a lot of people struggle with and although I am super religious myself, I do understand why people struggle with it. I just think it makes life a lot easier to think that if we pass the challenges this life throws at us, we can go to a better world or a place of peace. Religion is what saved me in my darkest hour, and I feel I have seen enough in my life to believe that someone is watching over me and guiding me in the right direction.

Self-improvement is one big part of leading a successful happy life. Some of the other parts to this I believe are hard work and having a *"no excuses"* attitude as I like to call it. It is all down to your decisions - no one else is to blame, just your choices, your life and it's up to you whether it's a success or not.

To live with this attitude, you get up early every day, work on yourself and then give the day your best shot every single time. You don't go in half-hearted and then tell everyone you can't be bothered. What a waste of a day or even months/years for some people. We get a limited time on this earth and so many people waste it just taking life for granted! Work hard at something, be energetic towards your day but have a laugh and make it fun along the way. Work with people who push you to achieve your best but can laugh with you and at you along the way. Every day in this world is a blessing - don't waste it.

Working hard doesn't mean ruining your family life. Be efficient, work as hard as you can while you're at work and then when you're done for the day, focus solely on what's going on at home. So many people say they work long hours and they're just not being efficient enough with their time. If *Jeff Bezos* can find time to have tea and clean the dishes at night, so can you.

So, there is a fine line between working hard and wasting time. Get up early, get all your jobs done for the day and do something that challenges you. Try to move your job or business forward every day and then find your cut off point. Then try as hard as you can to make the family time as good as possible and obviously don't forget to find the time for self-improvement tasks that make you feel great.

Be disciplined, you're not going to wake up feeling great every day no matter how positive you are, but it's just about keeping going. I wake up sore or with some sort of ache every day but still train. Why do I do this? Because when I feel like this it's probably that negative part of my mind trying to protect us and get back in control of our lives. Well, we don't need it unless it's stopping us from jumping off buildings or walking into a burning house - so don't listen to it! Just be consistent every day in your positive habits and give your best at them. It doesn't have to be perfect every day, most of the time it's just about showing up and trying. If you can teach your mind to just keep showing up, trying your best and facing every problem 7 days a week - I guarantee you you'll be one of the best and most successful people in this world because you'll have cracked the hardest bit. I don't bargain with my mind. If I don't feel like facing up to some problem or training, I start laughing to myself because I know from my life experience if I don't do it, it will cause even more problems. If I face it, I'll feel great and the rest of my day will be better. It will lead to less problems by facing it up to it now rather than delaying it and letting the problems build up. If you give your brain an inch with excuses it'll take a mile, you'll not just eat one cake you'll eat the full box and then it'll give you 100 reasons to why it's ok that you ate them. Just don't eat the first cake! On your road to success and self-improvement you have got to be really careful about your self-talk. It's something we all need to work hard on, and it links in a lot with your beliefs. When things go wrong, our fears and past experiences kick in in and our mind starts using old stories to back up that we're useless and can't do things. Unfortunately, no matter how much we improve - these thoughts are always going to creep into our subconscious mind when things go wrong or we're having a bad day. The trick is to learn to let them go by, to laugh at them and not focus on them. We need to replace these thoughts with some powerful self-talk like telling ourselves, *"just keep going"* and that, *"we've dealt with challenges before and we'll deal with them again."* One of my favourite quotes on this is from the book '*Feel the Fear and Do It Anyway*' by Susan Jeffers. She says, *"if we knew we could deal with anything that came our way, what would we have to fear? NOTHING."* All of our fears about a situation usually come from the thought that we can't deal with it not working out the way we want it to. When we look back at our lives, we've always dealt with everything that happened to us because we're still here, so tell yourself whatever happens you'll deal with it!

Studies have also shown that a negative thought is 4 times more powerful than a positive one and when spoken out loud it can be up to 7 times more powerful! So, when a negative thought pops up in your head don't at all costs even think of saying it out loud - let it go! Talking negative thoughts out loud is a common bad habit which makes the thought grow stronger and brings us down even further. This increases the chance of that bad thing occurring because we've planted that seed of thought so strongly in our brains. The mind is a powerful tool, it's so important that we stop it from working against us.

If you talk positives, your mind will listen to you and you'll feel positive. Our words and body language have a big impact on how we feel, so keep them both positive. Walking around with your head up and a smile on your face will lead to you feeling better and having more positive interactions with people because you look a nice, happy person even when you're having a hard day.

Also, the words and actions of others can have a massive impact on how we feel and our success in life.

One of the truest sayings goes, *"if your 5 best friends are millionaires, you'll be the sixth. If you surround yourself with 5 idiots, you'll be the sixth."* So, we must be very careful who we associate with and spend our time with. Their thoughts and opinions can easily become our own and their actions and habits usually do too. If you're unsuccessful or in a bad place and your friends are the same – reassess whether they are really enhancing your life and if need be, get rid of them. It is very hard to be positive around people who are negative. They can drag you down in ways you won't even realise. It can be draining to keep your mood up around these people and a complete waste of energy. That's why it's way better for you to just leave the friendship group. As hard as it is you've got to be honest with yourself and disciplined if you want a successful life. If you've not got the discipline to walk away from negative surroundings, don't blame the world for your unhappy life.

Don't get me wrong there are so many amazing loving, caring, kind, enthusiastic people in this world, but still there are twice as many negative individuals. As positive as a lot of people in this group will think they are, when you get into their skin you will find that they talk negatively about people, haven't faced their insecurities and they still blame the world for what has gone wrong in their lives. My challenge to you is to be different, be the type of person who gets up every morning, gives the world their best shot and is the bright spark in everyone's day. Be the person who everyone feels positive around but people know not to bring negativity to because if they do, you'll tell them straight and won't stand for it. Be the person who has a purpose, who does work for charity and truly loves their job. Be that success story that everyone loves to hear about and makes everyone else believe they can do it themselves. Be that person who's up early every morning trying their best, never letting their mind get the better of them. Live from your heart, your soul and not your ego. I hope this book and my story gives you something to think about and has shown you the incredible power of our mind if we don't train it and aren't careful what we feed it with. Also, how you can live an amazing, happy, successful life and not just from when you reach you goal - but the second you start to read this book. I hope it encourages you to make a difference in the world and be that positive change the world needs! Go and be the best possible version of you, the world needs you!

Go and get started now!

ACKNOWLEDGEMENTS

I would like to thank Matt Bacon and Adam Smith at LMD
Publications for doing a great job of publishing and editing this
book for me. Without Matt's help, this book would not have been
made possible.

Also, my sister Lucy Collins for the initial editing and helping me
to get my message across on paper. Thirdly, Robyn Sinclair for her
amazing photography skills that have made the front and back
covers look incredible.

I would like to say a big thank-you to my family, friends and clients
for giving me the energy and reason to fight when times got most
dark and for inspiring me to give everything I can to help end
suffering for as many people as possible.

<u>Helpful references for the reader</u>

Books:

Anthony Robbins - *'Awaken the Giant Within'*

Viktor Frankl - *'Man's Search for Meaning'*

James Clear - *'Atomic Habits: An Easy & Proven Way*

to Build Good Habits & Break Bad Ones'

Dale Carnegie - *'How to Win Friends and Influence People'*

Susan Jeffers - *'Feel the Fear and Do It Anyway.*

A little more about the author...

Who am I?

Not your average Joe!
I take your personal fitness goals seriously. I understand that losing weight and gaining muscle can be challenging, and our goal is to help you overcome hurdles and reach your goals. My services analyse your body type, BMI, and metabolism to create your individualized fitness plan.

Knowledgeable Training Expertise
With years of success and experience, I am capable of analysing your body and creating a fitness plan that will help you reach your goals. Most plans include healthy eating and exercise, to ensure the best results for our clients. I will work with you to keep you on track and motivated to reach your goals.

Mental awareness and stability
COVID-19 has taken its toll on all of us and I can offer qualified assistance to bring out your inner potential. There is always a helping hand and an open door to both clients and the public if alike whether you prefer face to face or anonymous call, I am here to help any stressors to lift the weight off your shoulders.

Visit **www.joecollinshealth.com** for more information.